INTRODUCTION

As early as 2008, I have had this magnificent idea of writing a book. It was a time when I was coming to an end of a ten year career as a solo Pediatrician. The practice of medicine was beginning to change   and insurance companies were beginning to dictate even more how we as physicians could practice medicine. I was not happy with these changes I saw taking place, especially in my field of pediatrics. Now here it is, January 2011 and I have finally figured out how I was going to approach all of what I want to say in several short guides for parents. I have had so many concerns that have compiled up over the years. Concerns so strong, I question myself often. Is the dream I have had as long as can remember being fulfilled? That dream is being an advocate for children; as a pediatrician.

As you know, as physicians, we take an oath, an oath that we promise to honor, and live by. An oath practiced by physicians swearing to practice medicine to the maximum and of course ethically. What does "ethically" really mean in the world of modern medicine? "Ethically" as defined by Webster, means "being in accordance with the accepted principles of right and wrong that govern the conduct of a profession.

It was May 1995, after what I thought were the most grueling four years of my life. I stood with my fellow classmates and recited the

Hippocratic Oath. From that day forth, I was set out to "cure" every child that set foot in my office. That is the reason I spent four years in medical school in addition to another three years specializing in pediatrics, right? I wanted to make this world a much better place for children. Did my other classmates have this same vision as a medical professional? Does the Hippocratic Oath still today, hold its meaning and value as it did when it was originally written and later updated in 1994 by Louis Lasagna?

THE HIPPOCRATIC OATH

"I swear to fulfill, to the best of my ability and judgment, this consent. I will respect the hard won scientific gains of those physicians in whose steps I walk and gladly share such knowledge as is mine with those who are to follow. I will apply, for the benefit of the sick, all measures that are required, avoiding those turn traps of over treatment and therapeutic nihilism. I will remember that there is an art to medicine as well as science, and that warmth, sympathy, and understanding may outweigh the surgeon's knife or chemist's drugs. I will be ashamed to say 'I know not,' nor will I fail to call on of my colleagues when the skills of another are needed for a patient's recovery. I will respect the privacy of my patients, for their problems are not disclosed to me that the world may know. Most especially must I treat with care the matters of life and death, if it is given to me to save a life, all thanks. But it may also be within my power to take a life. This awesome responsibility must be faced with great humbleness and awareness of my own frailty. Above all, I must not play with God. I will remember that I do not treat a fever chart, a cancerous growth, but a sick human being, whose illness may affect the person's family and economic stability. My responsibility includes these related problems, if I am to care adequately for the sick. I will prevent disease whenever I can, for prevention is preferable to cure. I will remember that I remain a member of society, with special obligations to all my fellow human beings, those sounds of mind and body as well as the infirm. If I violate this oath, may I enjoy life and art, respected while I live and remember with affliction thereafter. May I always act so as to preserve the finest traditions of my calling and may I long experience the joy of healing those who seek my help."

CHAPTER 1

UNDERSTANDING ATTENTION DEFICIT HYPERACTIVITY DISORDER (ADHD)

ADHD, as it is well known referred to, is a rapidly growing diagnosis among young children and adolescents worldwide. There are multiple drugs being manufactured just for this particular behavioral disorder. Why are we seeing so many cases of ADHD which has drastically increased over the last five to seven years? Why is it that three-fourths of the medications administered by the school nurse are stimulate medications? I not only speak professionally on the subject of ADHD, but I also speak from a parental point of view having a son myself diagnosed as having ADHD. So I can truly empathize with parents who are trying to understand this troubling disorder.

Attention deficit hyperactivity disorder, first of all is a terribly named disorder. Why is it called "attention deficit" when there is no deficit of attention? We are just use to thinking of an illness as resulting from a shortage of "something." People with thyroid disease are missing thyroid stimulating hormone. People with diabetes are lacking or missing the cells in the pancreas to attack the accumulation of sugar in the body. Attention deficit hyperactivity disorder does not seem to work as such. Recent evidence has suggested that children with ADHD have plenty of "attention." That's why they're able to play video games for hours, or get all lost in their music or legos, or devote endless attention to activities that they find interesting.

ADHD is really about the allocation of attention, being able to control their mental spotlight. The number one question I was always faced with as a physician from parents was, "what is the problem with children with ADHD?" Again, I found it useful to speak in allocation of attention when talking with parents dealing with ADHD children. What we should be wondering is where is the child's attention is being allocated? Is it where it needs to be to meet the demands of home, school, and society? Allocating one's attention appropriately for success in school requires willful control to turn away from a preferred activity and focus on an activity not as compelling or immediately rewarding.

Attention deficit hyperactivity disorder affects between 1.5 and 3.5 million school aged children in the United States, or an estimated 5% of all boys and 2% of all girls. Why it affects more boys than girls is still a mystery. Up to 60% of these children will continue to have symptoms of ADHD into their adulthood. According to the National Institutes of Health, more than a million children take prescription medication to control their hyperactive behavior. The estimated cost to schools is roughly $3 million. If as a child, you had ADHD, you might have had some symptoms of ADHD such as trouble reading that first paragraph in your lesson book without getting distracted. I'm sure your mind wondered off to a million other things you could've been doing rather than sitting there in a classroom.

I can remember as a child sitting in class focused on everything but what I was supposed to be focused on. When I wasn't interested in what was going on in the classroom, I became fidgety. Looking outside to see who was passing by, looking to see if other students were just as fidgety as I was. I remember oh so well being sent to the principal's office on multiple occasions because of my behavior. Was it ever suggested by the teacher or school principle that I might have ADHD and possibly needed to be on medication? My parents implemented other means of behavioral modifications; spankings, no television, or no after school activities until I could learn to behave in class. Almost everyone at some point exhibits signs of ADHD. We all get distracted. We all have trouble finishing our work or tasks. However, children with ADHD are, in general, less able to care for themselves, less able to communicate than children without ADHD of the same age.

The Diagnostic and Statistical Manuel of Mental Disorders, (DSM-IV), published by the American Psychiatric Association has a specific listing of behaviors that must be observed before a diagnosis of ADHD is made. Importantly, remember there are many reasons, other than ADHD, why children may exhibit the same behaviors of hyperactivity or a lack of attention. Infections, learning disabilities, or educational issues may mimic symptoms of ADHD. ADHD is a diagnosis of exclusion. On any given day, the symptoms of ADHD in a child may be absent, leading others to think that children can possibly control their behaviors. A definite diagnosis is difficult because there are no tests that can consistently diagnose ADHD. It is very important that attention deficit hyperactivity disorder is diagnosed by a healthcare professional that specializes in childhood behavioral disorders and is also familiar with the various behavioral disorders in children. Children are mistakenly being diagnosed with ADHD every day. Most kids with ADHD receive this diagnosis after a doctor takes a quick look at the child's behavior during an office visit. In some cases, it's very possible that there is actually nothing abnormal in the child's behavior at the time of the visit but a case of anxiety from being in a doctor's office and not knowing what to expect. Then there's the group of children who have been diagnosed with ADHD mistakenly because they are just simply a genius, no pun intended. These gifted children exhibit the same symptoms as children with ADHD. These are children with a greater intellectual capacity and creative ability than their peers. Gifted children tend to behave differently from their classmates and may be more precocious or hyperactive than the average child. Many of our public school systems are not trained to handle or be able to recognize a gifted child versus a non-gifted child. Is it possible that the medications used to treat ADHD symptoms can inhibit the intellectual curiosity and creativity in gifted children. For this reason alone, children definitely need a thorough evaluation of their symptoms and circumstances before any diagnosis or treatment is initiated. Below are just a few examples which differentiates ADHD and the "gifted" child, both which share similar symptoms.

ADHD

- Poor attention span in almost every situation.

- Easily gives up on tasks.

- Makes impulsive decisions and displays poor delay in gratification.

- Socially shy or inhibited.

- More active and restless than average.

- Have a hard time following rules.

- Failure to pay attention to details.

- Forgetting things that are needed to complete a task.

- Rarely follows directions completely or properly.

- Unable to sit still.

- Very talkative

- Leaving their seat when sitting is expected.

- Very impulsive to the point often making inappropriate comments.

- Shouts out answers before a question is finished.

- Behavior is such that it may put others in danger.

GIFTED

- Easily bored, poor attention span, and daydreams only in specific situations.

- Gets bored by tasks they think are irrelevant.

- Judgment often lags behind and the development of their intellect.

- Socially intense and engages in power struggles with those in authority.

- Have high activity levels only in certain situations.

- Questions rules, customs, and traditions.

CHAPTER 2

WHAT CAUSES ADHD

The cause of ADHD is still unclear although millions of children have been diagnosed with this behavioral disorder and are currently receiving treatment. It has been predicted though, that the cause of ADHD is related to certain receptors in the brain that respond to a neurotransmitter called dopamine. It's believed dopamine is being produced at decreased levels than normal in the brain. This defect in dopamine production occurs in the anterior frontal cortex of the brain. The anterior frontal cortex area is associated with cognitive processes such as focusing and attention. Evidence has also shown that children who were born weighing less than 1500g (3.3 lbs) or who had birth complications may be more prone to ADHD. There are still many other factors which are being investigated today to find out what role pregnancy complications possibly may play in ADHD. Could exposure to certain environmental factors be a contributor?

ENVIROMENTAL FACTORS POSSIBLY CAUSING ADHD:

- Toxins (lead)
- Drugs (alcohol/drugs)
- Excessive viewing of the television
- Food allergies
- Excess sugar
- Poor home life
- Poor schools

There has been an amazingly increase in evidence suggesting that ADHD is an inherited condition. If one identical twin has symptoms of ADHD, the other twin has a 75-92% chance of sharing the same trait. Children with ADHD are also likely to have one close relative who also has it. One-third of all fathers who had ADHD when younger have children who have ADHD as well. Adoption studies have proved more evidence of a genetic link to ADHD than adoptive relatives of children with ADHD. Past studies have shown that boys with ADHD tend to have brains that are more symmetrical in shape. It has been identified that three structures in the brains of boys with ADHD were smaller than in boys without ADHD of the same age. Those structures of the brain are the pre-frontal cortex, caudate nucleus, and globus pallidus. The prefrontal brain is considered the command center while the caudate nucleus and globus pallidus translate commands into the action.

With the advancement in technology, new studies demonstrate

that not only are some of the structures different as I mentioned earlier, but the brain may use these areas differently. By brain scan, researchers have noticed that boys with ADHD have an abnormal increase of activity in two structures of the frontal lobe and striate areas below it. These areas work to control voluntary action. The boys with ADHD were working harder to control their impulses than on boys without ADHD. Once given a stimulate drug, which is the first line of treatment used in children with ADHD, this abnormal activity slowed down. This kind of effect was not seen in the non-ADHD boys. Although the brain scan, known as functional Magnetic Resonance Image; MRI, is quite expensive; costing about $1700, it may provide a more accurate way to diagnose attention deficit hyperactivity disorder properly.

CHAPTER 3

TREATMENT

Medications have been the first line of treatment for ADHD in more children. We all know that the medications to treat this disorder have side effects and risks like any other medications. Here I will list most of the side effects of these medications used in the treatment of ADHD. With the abundance of medications on the market now, it is normal that parents of children with ADHD will find it challenging to select a medication that will suit their child. A stimulate, such as Ritalin, is known to improve a child's ability to control their impulses, concentration, help them completing their tasks and to plan ahead. Just keep in mind that these stimulates do not address all of the symptoms associated with ADHD, such as forgetfulness, emotional problems, relationship problems and organization. It is important that besides the medications, parents who have children with ADHD also help them make lifestyle changes, such as sleep, eating a more healthier diet, and regular exercise.

Stimulates are the most common medications prescribed by physicians in treating ADHD today. These drugs have a long track record. Some of the popular stimulates are Ritalin, Adderral, and Concerta just to name a few. They work by increasing the dopamine levels in the brain. Remember, children diagnosed with ADHD have decreased levels of dopamine production in the brain. Some of the common side effects of these stimulates are the tendency to become socially withdrawn, rigid, talkative, and listless. Some of the non-stimulates prescribed are Strattera, high blood pressure medications, and atypical antidepressants. Strattera works by boosting the levels of a brain chemical called norepinepherine. Norepiephrine works alongside epinephrine/adrenaline to give the body sudden energy in times of stress, known as "flight or fight" response. The various stimulates are available in long and short acting dosages. The effects of the long acting or extended release stimulates could last for 8-10 hrs and are taken once daily. The shorter acting stimulates are taken 2-3 times per day. The high blood pressure medications used are known to be effective in targeting hyperactivity, aggression, and impulsivity. The more common "high blood pressure" medications used for ADHD are clonipine and guanfacine; but physicians may choose others. Antidepressants help because they target several other neurotransmitters in the brain of individuals with ADHD.

The most alarming side effects of stimulates are their addictive properties. Two of the most common of these stimulates thought to lead to addiction, are Adderall and Concerta in the teenage and young adult population. University students use these two particular drugs as recreational drugs to boost their grades, improve athletic performance, and it is very popular among females to aid in losing weight. As one gets addicted, the side effects take a turn for the worse, especially among non-ADHD patients.

SIDE EFFECTS OF STIMULATE MEDICATIONS

RITALIN

- Headaches
- Loss of appetite
- Stunts the growth of children
- Drowsiness
- Nervousness
- Hair loss
- Anemia
- Changes in liver function
- Chest pains
- Heart palpitations
- Fainting
- Hallucinations

CONCERTA

- Headaches
- Upper respiratory infections
- Loss of appetite in up to 25% of patients
- Dry mouth
- Tics (uncontrolled movements)
- Painful menstrual periods
- Abdominal pain
- Suicidal thoughts
- Chest tightness
- Shortness of breath.

ADDERALL

- Headaches
- Weight loss due to loss of appetite
- Dry mouth
- Chest tightness
- Stomach pains
- Increase in blood pressure
- Nausea
- Vomiting
- Increased heart rate
- Upper respiratory infections
- Fever

- Heartburn
- Emotional changes.

CLONIDINE

- Dry mouth
- Fatigue
- Constipation
- Vomiting
- Lightheadedness
- Fainting
- Chest pains
- Fast or slow heart rate
- Depression
- Anxiety
- Congestive heart failure
- Difficulty breathing.

STRATTERA

- Stomach aches
- Vomiting
- Nausea
- Loss of appetite
- Dry mouth
- dizziness,
- difficulty sleeping
- menstrual cycle change
- mood changes weight loss
- unusual heart beat
- Headaches
- and blurred vision

Unfortunattely, Straterra has been linked to heart failure and suicide. Eli Lily, the makers of Straterra, warned doctors that Straterra, had caused several liver injuries in several patients. When this finding was announced, Eli Lily and two other pharmaceutical companies lose a total of $30 billion in stock volume.

CHAPTER 4

THE OVERDIAGNOSING OF ADHD

Is ADHD being over diagnosed? I still question this after 15 years of practicing pediatrics. Within recent years, a phenomenon has taken place within the school system in the United States which involves the classification of millions of children labeled with the behavioral disorder, attention deficit hyperactivity disorder; ADHD as we know it. For an employer, parent, counselor, educator and even physicians of someone meeting the specified criteria for an ADHD diagnosis, the right interactions and the sustaining of attention can be frustrating. The increasing numbers of diagnoses lead many to question the validity of many of these classifications. When working in the field of human services or education, the contact with those that exhibit behaviors similar or in line to the criteria for ADHD is highly noted. It has been very easy to classify someone with ADHD in an attempt to normalize behaviors or to provide explanations as to why a child does not fit into a certain mold, rather strategizing or coping with the frustrating situations. The controversy over this diagnosis category has been broadened due to further research about the behavioral disorder in relation to normal development of kids.

Many researchers are even questioning now, based on lack of sufficient evidence, whether ADHD is even an authentic psychiatric disorder. Did you know that it has been proposed that the diagnosis of ADHD has no grounds as more than grouping of behaviors, rather than a psychological disorder that can be treated and maintained with the use of medication? The biggest controversial question to date is if there are grounds for the medical diagnosis. Why are so many kids being treated with aggressive stimulates? You will be shocked at the most formulated answers to these questions involving the government and the pharmaceutical companies.

It is very interesting to note that ADHD, as a major disorder of childhood behavioral and/or cognitive abilities, is an overwhelming American problem compared to any other society within the world. The American fixation on finding quick solutions for difficult solutions and for difficult situations may be to blame. Although the difficulty of managing behaviors of extreme inattention and hyperactivity occur within the home, the largest push for solutions to these behaviors occurs within the academic settings. For a teacher, it could be very frustrating to have to continually redirect one specific child while attempting to give that same attention to 30 or 40 students, but does that justify medicating for the sake of ease over the sake of the child's well being? Did you know that with the implementation of new educational acts and funding, schools are even able to receive benefits; monies for each student who is medically diagnosed with ADHD and most of these assessments of ADHD in the schools, are ironically conducted by school board employed educational psychologists. Knowing that fact, I recommend to always have your child evaluated by your personal physician or another qualified medical personnel NOT associated within the school system. Could ADHD be a diagnosis of convenience? Psychiatry made a list of the most common symptoms of emotional discomforts of kids; those which bothered the teachers and parents the most and termed them a "disease". Twenty five years of research, not deserving of the term actually "research", has failed to validate ADHD as a disease.

Currently over 7 million kids in America are taking stimulate drugs for ADHD, most commonly the brain disabling narcotics Ritalin, Concerta, or Strattera just to name a few. In the U.K., the latest figures show about 500,000 prescriptions for stimulates for under age 16. Australia has also shown over 50,000 kids who are currently using drugs for ADHD and these numbers are rapidly rising. Many parents are unaware that Ritalin is a class II narcotic, which has a chemical composition and function similar to both amphetamines ("speed") and cocaine. Ritalin is addictive and subject to severe withdrawal symptoms. Some of these side effects as discussed earlier, can be permanent including growth stunting, brain atrophy, loss of muscular control, loss of self regard, seizures, spasms, and even sudden death. Although you may be told that these side effects are "rare", they can still occur. So why are medical practioners recommending to parents that they give medication as first line treatment to their children? Why are schools recommending to parents to get their child assessed for ADHD opposed to implementing some common behavior modification techniques first? Is medication really needed in order for children to pay attention in class? Psychologists and behavioral scientists say that attention is a form of consciousness so it can not be observed. Recall what ADHD stands for; attention deficit hyperactivity disorder. But there is no real deficit of attention.

Millions of kids are hit with this diagnosis of ADHD. Sometimes, it seems that the kids who have not been diagnosed with ADHD might just start feeling left out. Who knows, maybe they too will start acting out just to get some attention. Ten percent of all kids between the ages of 4-17 years old were diagnosed with ADHD in 2007. That is 5.4 million kids overall; up from 4.4 million in 2003. A 22% rise according to the U.S Center for Disease Control and Prevention survey. The biggest boost has been in the Hispanic children, where there has been an increase of 53% diagnosed with ADHD. There has also been an alarming number in older kids between the ages of 15-17 years old. This increase in kids 15-17 yr age group is disturbing because it has been hypothesized that many of them may simply fake the condition simply to get their hands on the stimulate medications. There are even online communities providing tips to these teens on faking ADHD to get the stimulate medication. Next time you are sitting at your computer, goggle "fake ADHD" and see the numerous results that will pop up.

The fact is, the kids who are not faking it may not have ADHD, because the problem in many cases is not with the child, it is with the teachers and doctors and even the parents who are just as quick to diagnose a disruptive child as an ADHD situation. Two recent studies found that millions of American children may have been misdiagnosed simply because they are younger and are less mature than their classmates, or just simply "gifted". Researchers even looked at kids and ADHD diagnoses and arranged these kids by birthdates. The findings were that the youngest kid in any given kindergarten classroom was about 60% more likely to be diagnosed with ADHD than the oldest kid in the same classroom.

Behavior modification should always be considered and tried first before jumping to the conclusion and tagging a child with ADHD. Behavior modification, good diet, and exercise are the real answers in my opinion. Do not be quick to medicate a child that is more than likely gifted with a high IQ or struggling with learning disabilities. More times than not, a highly intelligent child is not being challenged in the classroom and will act out in some way. They will either be the class clown or the class bully.

ADHD is in fact very difficult to diagnose as personalities and behaviors differ from one person to another. When kids are growing and forming these different behavioral traits, they often tend to go through phases. These phases can make it extremely difficult to determine if a child is hyperactive. When assessing a child in order to determine if they truly do have ADHD or not, several critical questions to consider first are listed below:

- Does the child's behavior occur in different settings?
- Is the behavior temporary or a continual situation?

- Does the child's behavior occur more often than not, in children of the same age?
- Is the behavior long term, excessive, or pervasive to others?

Many physicians will diagnose a child with ADHD and prescribe medications even if the child does not completely fit the profile of an ADHD child because the school can no longer deal with the behavior or the parents have become frustrated; especially if there are other children in the household. Other conditions to consider before making an ADHD diagnosis are:

- Emotional problems
- Allergies
- Scholastic problems
- Anxiety
- Depression
- Ear infections/hearing loss

CHAPTER 5

INCENTIVES FOR A DIAGNOSIS OF ADHD

In the United States alone, psychiatrists, doctors, and Eli Lily are all cashing in on the drugging of both children and adults for ADHD and ADD which are both diagnoses by exclusion as mentioned earlier. The insidious relationship between the American Psychiatric Association, FDA, and the drug industries are one of the biggest crimes in the history of our country. The pharmaceutical industry has so much money to throw around; they can pretty much do whatever they want with no accountability. It was against the law for the drug industry to directly advertise prescription drugs to the public. Well it appears; the pharmaceutical industry has paid and lobbied their way to have that law changed, because we continuously keep getting direct advertisements on television, radio, and magazine ads. These advertisements have tremendously increased profits among pharmaceutical companies.

Now days, all you get on television are "do you suffer from adult ADD or ADHD? Ask your doctor if Strattera is right for you". Now they are targeting adults as well as children. It's getting to the point where consumers are telling their doctor what prescriptions they need, when it should be the other way around. Because of this, direct to consumer advertising of prescription medications should be banned. The FDA's not doing anything about it; is it because they get so much money from the drug industry? Why doesn't the DEA step in? The risks, dangers, and deaths from these stimulate medications have been exposed. Since the dangers of psycho-stimulates have been exposed, the drug industry still needs a way to continue cashing in on ADHD and ADD. This is why Strattera, the new heavily advertised drug has been advertised as the new non-stimulate drug. Very clever wouldn't you say? Federal health officials are preparing stronger warnings for some antidepressants used in children after new analyses back a possible link to suicide. I am no chemist but when you compare antidepressants and Strattera, they look very similar in their chemical makeup. I sure hope we don't find out the hard way that the name of the drug was changed with minor chemical makeup changes only to continue the profits rolling in at the expense of our children.

Let me take you inside a little closer at the Federal Disability Programs. Congress created Supplemental Security Income (SSI) in 1974 to aid the aged, blind, and severely physically disabled, such as children with Downs Syndrome and Cerebral Palsy, yet one-half of today's SSI recipients are children diagnosed with ADHD and bipolar disorder. In 1990, only 8% of children received SSI funds for behavioral issues. By 2009, that percentage skyrocketed to 53% and even more shocking than that, children under 5 years of age are the fastest growing segment of this steep. The most disturbing aspect of all of these government incentives to lower income families is it discourages healthy alternatives. It is one of those unintended consequences of a government program which was started with the best intentions; to help the poorest of the poor families get adequate treatment for their "disabled" child.

The Boston Globe ran an in-depth investigation about some of these consequences which included rampant diagnosing of very young children and the over prescribing of medication. Many cash strapped parents believe that if they can muster the necessary medical records, their children have a shot at these benefits, even if it does carry the stigma of the word "disabled." The SSI program, was a program designed to help only a small minority of children; those with serious health or mental disabilities. This SSI program is now serving approximately 53% of the 1.2 million of children who actually qualify for the programs benefits. Are you curious as to know what the number one diagnosis is of children receiving these SSI benefits? Of course, the number one diagnosis is attention deficit hyperactivity disorder; ADHD. With over 90% of my pediatric population being from the underserved population and receiving Government assistance, hundreds of these disability applications came through my office yearly and I refused to fill out hundreds as well. Parents were merely seeking that supplemental check for their "disabled" child.

Now, another disturbing part of the program seems to be the mandate by the federal governmental offices who administer this program. In order for a child to be considered disabled, the child is required to be on psychiatric medications regardless whether the parent wants them to or not. In one instance with a friend of mine who was seriously questioning whether her boys needed to be on stimulate meds or not, saw firsthand how this "incentive" program worked. I evaluated both of her boys in my office and suggested behavioral modification methods first and to then possibly seek a psychologist for a more thorough evaluation before considering any medications. She never liked the sound of medication anyway. She also believed that too many of today's children are being "over medicated" with stimulate medications and she did not want this for her boys; although other clinicians that had seen the boys were labeling them with diagnoses such as, oppositional defiant disorder, depression and ADHD. As medical bills started piling up, friends suggested to her to seek help through the SSI office. Eventually, she did go ahead with the suggestion. She then went ahead and submitted the appropriate applications for disability. During this time she was applying, both boys were not on any type of medication and both applications rejected. One year later, school officials persuaded her to at least let her 14 year old son try the drug for his impulsiveness. Within weeks after she had reapplied for the SSI benefits, which she had previously been denied, she was approved. Did you catch what the keyword for SSI approval was? Of course, it was the medication that got that stamp of "approval" that got this mother SSI benefits for her son.

Why do poor parents do it? It merely comes down to the basic economics. You get money from the government if your child is labeled as "disabled." SSI payments can be a lifetime in a bad economy and they beat welfare checks in every way. In many northeast states, a parent with two children; welfare pays a maximum of about $600.00 per month. If just one of those two kids is approved for SSI benefits, the total government benefits can be twice as much. Are you getting this picture on how the government can be involved in "over medicating" children? Of course the reality is that most children, who have ADHD, are nowhere close to the classic definition of "disabled." Even mental disorders can be treated as effectively with psychotherapy and behavioral modifications as well as they can with psychiatric medications. The fall back with behavioral modification or any other therapy that does not involve medications is that, there is no monetary gain from the SSI office. So parents are being caught up in an unintended reward situation where if they agree to medicate their child, they can suddenly qualify for more money from the government. This definitely explains the discrepancy in the diagnosis of children with ADHD; the poorer that are on Medicaid, have a larger percentage of ADHD diagnoses.

Now I will speak on the parallel to pharmaceutical companies' involvement along with the government programs. While SSI payouts for behavioral issues sky rocketed since the 90's, so have drug profits. Pharmaceutical sales shot up from $40 billion in 1990 to $234 billion in 2008. The industry's vast frontal network of mental health advocates lobby at every opportunity for government backing of their child medicating campaign. The common growing issues of frustrations, defiance's, and mood swings, and spontaneity have been redefined into psychiatric "disorders." With some 15 million children reportedly having "learning disabilities," this just points to the failure with the schools, not the students. Not to stray from the main subject here, but with childhood obesity at a high, did you know there is a push now on screening more children for high cholesterol and to put them on high cholesterol medications? I have dealt with a lot of over weight kids in my practice where they have had high cholesterol levels. I have never in my 15 year career had to put a child on medication to bring the cholesterol levels down to normal. The only thing I had to do was to create a healthier diet and encourage exercise; a form of behavior modification.

The drug industry has become the biggest defrauders of the federal government. The drug industry has paid out nearly $20 billion in penalties over the past 2 decades for violations of the False Claims Act. More than half of these fines were paid by just four of the many drug companies that exist today. Pfizer alone, recently as 2009, paid out the largest criminal fine in the United States. This fine was $1.2 billion for illegally promoting drugs that were NOT approved for what it was claimed to treat; this action is called 'illegal off label promotion'. The interesting thing is that, of that $20 billion, three-quarters of it has just been in the last five years. What we are seeing here is an escalation of well organized criminal and other kinds of legal-illegal activity by the pharmaceutical companies, the same companies that are manufacturing drugs for our kids. My purpose of telling you all about these activities of pharmaceutical companies is not to destroy their reputation or credibility. I am simply, as a physician, allowing you to get a real glimpse and I do mean glimpse, as to what goes on behind the scenes. We usually only see or hear about such incidences on television shows such as 20/20 or Dateline after some sort of investigation following a tragic event. Keep in mind that these are companies that are medicating your children. Do they have the safety of human beings at best interest or is their best interest in the profits that they can generate at the expense of humans; children in this case.

CHAPTER 6

BEHAVIOR MODIFICATION TECHNIQUES

Behavior therapy includes interventions that are focused on modifying the social and physical environment of a child to alter behavior. Behavior modification has not always shown to be effective, but it's definitely worth trying before subjecting children to dangerous medications. So let's keep an open mind here. The same dose of Ritalin or any stimulate medication used in treating ADHD, will not have the same effect on every child, so do not expect behavior modification to either. Behavior modification will vary and you must adjust any program to suit any particular child. Behavior modification therapy alone may not be what helps with a child diagnosed with ADHD but if medication is part of a child's regime, behavior modification could possibly allow for a child to take a lesser dose; "two heads are better than one." While implementing the behavior therapy, keep in mind the following aspects:

1) **Non-competitive Aspect:** Children with ADHD are often not able to cope or benefit from competitive incentives such as "the first one finished gets the cupcake." Try not to involve them in such games.

2) **Accommodations to tasks and assignment:** As we are well aware, ADHD children naturally struggle with attention and often need more time to perform tasks. They may not be able to cope with the amount and level of homework that other children are able to do. They will need special accommodations for tasks and assignments to keep them motivated and avoid frustration. Small breaks in between study subjects can help.

3) Focus on teaching ADHD children a set of skills to replace "bad" behavior. "Regular" children are able to learn new skills on their own when they are told a certain behavior is wrong. Children with ADHD have difficulty with this. They need to be taught alternative skills to replace problem behaviors. For example, if your child has a tendency to misbehave at the diner table, they need to be taught different table manners and given an opportunity to practice good manners.

4) **Modify the Environment:** Children with ADHD study and learn better with small modifications in the environment. The desk or study table must be free of any distracting objects. They must sit away from the window or door. Some kids even work better with ear plugs or ear muffs on. Hey, keep in mind, as oddly as it may seem, do what works. My son would sometimes do his homework in his clothes closet. Whatever works for your child, flow with it.

5) **Visual Representation of Rules and Instructions:** Children with ADHD find it difficult to process and remember verbal instruction. It is much easier if the instructions are represented by a symbol or

picture. For older children, writing a list of chores or reminders down on a piece of paper is good.

6) **Bigger Rewards and Frequently Rotated:** When a child does something good, reward his/her behavior. For a "regular" child, the words "very good" may be sufficient, but a child with ADHD needs something tangible and bigger to keep motivation high. Remember to frequently rotate the rewards to make sure that they do not get bored with any one particular reward.

7) **Consequences Must Be Fast, Frequent, and High Magnitude:** When children engage in problem behaviors, the consequences need to be of a higher magnitude. The consequences must be delivered quickly and must be whenever the problem happens.

8) **Prepare Children for Change in Consequences:** A lot of children do not behave the right way because they do not clearly understand the change in circumstances or the expected behavior. For example, the child moving in from the playground into the classroom may not realize that "fun" time has ended and it is now "study" time; time to sit still. It is always good to go over the expectations of classroom time BEFORE the change in activity.

AFTER SCHOOL ACTIVITIES

The first step in choosing the right after school activity for your child is to first understand how ADHD affects him/her. Is your child interested in sports? Are they turned off from the fierce competition or does he/she find it hard to get along with teammates? For a child with ADHD, physical exercise is always beneficial. Exercise takes up that extra energy and helps stimulate the brain. Team activity teaches your child social skills and discipline. But if he/she shies away from team sports, you may want to look into some other types of activities such as swimming, dancing, cycling, or gymnastics. Importantly, find out what your child is interested in doing. Acting classes are a wonderful form of creative exercise. It can provide your child with ample opportunity to develop social skills. The options are unlimited in finding an activity suitable for your child. You just have to find out what interests your child. Make sure to monitor the progress periodically. If you feel that there is no progress, you may want to change the activity.